THE ART OF RUCKING - FM TAOR-01

First Edition

Author: Ken Schafer, in collaboration with Michael Glover

Editor: ChatGPT

Website: www.healthysexualitywithken.com

About Me: www.kenschafer.info

Email: contact@healthysexualitywithken.com

© 2024 Ken Schafer

FOREWORD

This book is a product of a collaboration between myself (Ken Schafer) and Michael Glover, founder of **The Art of Rucking**. We connected on TikTok, of all places. Once connected, we soon realized we had a lot in common, including the fact that we both had been interviewed on the Resisting Beta podcast. Realizing that we could accomplish more working together than we could individually, we got to work.

Michael Glover spent three years as an infantryman in the US Army. He is currently in the Army National Guard, supporting the 19th Special Forces Group, and works as a Federal Police Officer. Michael has 10 years of personal training experience. He used his experiences as a personal trainer and as an infantryman to develop The Art of Rucking.

I (Ken Schafer) spent 10 years on active duty with the US Army and 4 years in the Massachusetts Army National Guard. A few years ago, I picked up rucking as a hobby. I also have a degree in Exercise Science and various credentials as a running coach. I trained personally with Dr. Nicholas Romanov, who developed the Pose Method of Running.

You can find us at the following websites.

- Michael Glover - www.theartofrucking.com

- Ken Schafer - www.healthysexuality.com and www.kenschafer.info

You can contact us at the following emails.

- Michael Glover - theartofrucking@gmail.com
- Ken Schafer - contact@healthysexuality.com

If you want to learn about rucking, this is the place. Now, let's get started.

DEDICATION

Dedicated to all the men and women who sacrifice to serve the greater good.

TABLE OF CONTENTS

CHAPTER ONE

Introduction to Rucking

DEFINITION OF RUCKING

Rucking is military-style hiking. What does that mean exactly? The term rucking comes from the term "rucksack," which military personnel call their backpacks. Soldiers and Marines will often train by walking or hiking long distances wearing their loaded rucksacks. This type of training is referred to as "rucking."

So you may wonder if rucking is walking or hiking wearing a rucksack. How is this different from hiking? The answer is very little. Here are some differences as I see them. Others may disagree, but that's okay. These differences are not very important.

Generally, soldiers and Marines will be carrying a weapon. So, unlike hiking, their hands are not free to carry walking sticks. This can make rucking more challenging on difficult terrain. If you are a civilian and wish to carry a walking stick, carry one, but it's a luxury that those in the military do not have.

Usually, the packs are heavier in rucking. Soldiers and Marines often carry very heavy loads in combat, so they will train with heavy loads when rucking. This is not a requirement for rucking, especially for beginners, but it's something to keep in mind as you gain experience and become fitter.

Often, rucking is done with a military rucksack. Again, this is not a requirement, but many people like to stick with the military roots of rucking and training with surplus military gear.

The footwear that many people prefer to ruck in are military-style boots. As with everything I've already mentioned, this is not a requirement. If you are training for the military, I would encourage you to wear military footwear, but if you are a civilian rucking for health and fitness, wear whatever footgear works best for you.

BENEFITS OF RUCKING

What are the benefits of rucking? There are many. Some are obvious, and others may be more esoteric and personal.

Exercise: The first and most obvious benefit is health and fitness. Rucking is a relatively low-impact form of aerobic exercise. The great thing about rucking is that you can adjust the exercise to challenge yourself appropriately. You can adjust both the weight in your pack and your pace to meet your needs.

There is no question you can use rucking to become very fit. While I wouldn't recommend using rucking as your only form of exercise, it can be a part of a more comprehensive fitness program. However, it's fine if you only want to ruck for fitness. It will still greatly benefit your health and fitness.

Mental Toughness: Mental toughness has many facets, but one element is resilience. Endurance exercises, like rucking, often involve pushing through physical and mental discomfort. Learning to cope with this discomfort and continue despite it helps build resilience, a key component of mental toughness. Mental toughness is about becoming comfortable with discomfort, and rucking can be a way to introduce discomfort into your life. Over time, if you push through the discomfort, it won't bother you.

Getting out into nature: Not everyone loves to get out into nature, but this is one of my favorite perks of rucking. Living in New England in the US, I can easily jump on one of the hundreds of trail networks. This allowed me to disappear into the forest, away from the noise of my suburban neighborhood, and soak in the flora and fauna. It is not uncommon for me to trip over a deer and even an occasional bear. Fortunately, the bears in New England are not very aggressive.

Otherwise, I wouldn't be here to write this book.

Mediation: As a lifelong runner, I've always found running to be very meditative. Once you get into the rhythm, it's possible to enter a state of mental relaxation. The same thing can happen with cycling, rowing, and other activities where you perform the same motion repeatedly. Rucking is no different. Once you get into the rhythm, you focus inward and use it as a form of meditation.

Self-Reflection: Everyone can benefit from looking inward and asking themselves questions designed to challenge the status quo. Here are some questions I ask myself while rucking alone with my thoughts.

- How can I do better?
- How could I have handled that situation in a more positive way?
- What is getting in the way of me being the best version of myself?
- What are my weaknesses, and how can I address them?
- How do I contribute to my problems?

Clearly, the list of points to ponder is endless, but the idea is to figure out what you can do to improve yourself and your life by asking yourself some questions. Sometimes, uncomfortable questions.

Comradeship: If you are fortunate enough to have friends to train with, rucking can be a great way and a good time to build group cohesion and comradery. So many people, mostly men, do not have any close friends. Friends are essential to good mental health, If you want a better life build friendships. Rucking can help bring people, particularly men, together, to share common interests, and build friendships.

APPLICATIONS OF RUCKING IN MILITARY AND CIVILIAN SCENARIOS

There are probably many applications of rucking I've never thought of, but here are a few. Clearly, any activity that requires you to walk, especially under load, is a practical application of rucking.

Preparation for the military: If you are getting ready to join the military, I highly recommend that you get your body ready for the rigors of military life before entering the service. This is especially true if you are joining the Army or Marines in a combat-related specialty. Believe me, it's worth the effort.

Soldiers and Marines often have to ruck with very heavy loads all day. Then, if they are lucky, they will get a couple of hours of sleep, go on a mission, and then do it all over again the next day. They will do this often for weeks and even months at a time. If you don't prepare your body for that kind of strain, you will likely end up with long-term injuries.

Preparation for hiking: I love hitting the tails and getting out into nature. By rucking regularly, my body is more than prepared to deal with the challenges of hiking. Hiking is generally done at a more leisurely pace over a longer distance. If you ruck regularly, you will find that hiking will not be as challenging.

Prepping: In prepping and survivalist communities, there is a lot of discussion about "bugging out." Often, the discussions revolve around what you could take in a backpack if you had to hike to a safer location. I'm sure some readers just rolled their eyes. However, rucking can prepare you for a bug-out scenario if you are into preparedness.

The unfortunate reality is that many preppers I know are so focused on optimizing their gear and supplies that they neglect preparing their bodies for the physical demands of a disaster scenario. In a disaster scenario, a sound mind and body are your most important assets.

HOW TO GET STARTED

Variables

Four main variables determine the difficulty level in rucking load, speed, technique, and terrain.

Load

The most obvious variable is the load or weight you carry. Most civilians will train and compete with 20 to 45 lbs. People training for military applications will often train with 60 or more pounds. However, it's not just about the actual weight in your pack but also how it is distributed. The most efficient way to distribute the weight is close to your body and up near your shoulders. If you center the weight at the bottom of your pack and let it shift away from your body, you will have to work harder to walk/hike/run/ruck due to very well-understood laws of physics.

Assuming the weight is distributed properly, you can consider what your pack's actual weight should be for you. I encourage you to consider the weight as a percentage of your body weight. With some training, most people will quickly become comfortable with about 25 percent of their body weight. After that point, improvements will be more incremental. Again, everyone is different, and your experiences may vary.

Speed

How fast you walk is just as important as the weight you carry. Speed will be the most challenging aspect of your training if you are interested in competitions. For competitions and military training, 4 miles/hr is considered the standard for speed. That doesn't mean four mph has to be your goal. Your goals are entirely up to you.

Unfortunately, walking at 4 to 5 miles/hr requires practice because it is not a natural pace for a walking gait. At that speed, it's a toss-up whether it's more efficient to walk or jog. Fast walking will generally be easier for taller people than it is for shorter people.

If your goal is to ruck at 4 to 5 miles/hr, start with light loads and develop your speed-walking technique first. After achieving your desired pace, go up in weight. Again, your goals are to you. In fact, if your goal is to prepare for backpacking, you may want to focus on heavier loads at a slower pace.

Running with a ruck should be considered advanced training and not for beginners. If you are going to do this, it is vitally important that you start out with good running technique. If you have any problems with pain when you run, absolutely do not run with a ruck until you get your running technique problems sorted out. Ultimately, most of the pain associated with running is due to poor running technique.

Technique

Just like with running, the biggest problem I see with the rucking technique is overstriding. Many people mistakenly think that increasing their stride length will make them walk or run faster. Unfortunately, they have it backward. The faster you walk and run, the longer your stride will be. Stride length is a function of speed.

17

Speed is not a function of stride length. You should always put your foot down as close to your center of gravity as possible.

Terrain

Terrain will significantly affect your speed. As a short, late middle-aged man with a 60-pound pack, I can usually train at four mph or faster on flat ground with good footing. The area in which I live is quite hilly, though. As soon as I hit the hills, my speed is reduced to usually around 3.0 to 3.5 mph. Of course, it depends on the slope and length of the hills. Adjust your expectations accordingly.

Helpful Rules of Thumb

Here are some helpful rules of thumb about how these variables will affect your rucking. In my personal experience, these are pretty much correct. (See link to the article below)

- Every one percent of your body weight makes you six seconds slower per mile.

- Ten percent grade incline cuts your speed in half.

- Going up slows you down twice as much as going down speeds you up.

Original article - 5 RUN/RUCK TRAINING THUMB RULES YOU CAN USE. - **https://mtntactical.com/knowledge/5-runruck-training-thumb-rules-you-can-use/**

How To Get Started

For the purposes of this article, I'm going to assume you are generally healthy and can walk briskly without issues. If that's not the case, you are probably not ready to start rucking. Please contact me or Michael for for a more suitable training plan. See the forward for our contact info.

Pick a Course

As a beginner, it is better to pick a flat course. Generally, you want a course that you can finish within 60 minutes. For most people, three (3) to five (5) Km (2 to 3 miles) is a good distance to start with. Also, make sure the course has good footing and is safe.

Get a Good Rucking Pack

You will need a decent pack, especially as you increase your weight. Check out How to Build an Inexpensive Rucking Pack.

Start Rucking

Start with a very light pack. I suggest no more than 10 percent of your body weight. It's okay to start with less. Focus on walking briskly with proper technique and achieving your desired speed.

Incremental Improvement

Each week, or when you feel ready, add no more than 5 to 10 percent of your body weight to your pack. Less weight is fine. After adding the weight, focus again on waking briskly with good form. Don't add weight if you cannot maintain your desired speed and distance. Keep doing this until you reach your goal weight or 25 percent of your body weight, whichever comes first.

Time to Think about More Advanced Training.

Once you are rucking with 25 percent of your body weight, it's time to consider a more advanced program in which the weight, speed, distance, and terrain vary from workout to workout. Of course, some people want to keep things simple, which is absolutely fine.

How Far and How Much Time?

For beginners, start with distances you can cover in 30 to 60 minutes. As you get fitter and faster, you can increase the distance.

How Often?

I recommend 2 to 4 times a week for beginners. You need more recovery time if you feel burnt out, tired, or sore during most of your workouts. Cut back on the number of workouts for more recovery time. If you feel fresh during most of your workouts, consider doing them more often.

How Fast?

This will vary a lot from person to person. Start with light weights at a comfortable pace. When you are ready, focus on increasing the speed. The faster you go, the more technique matters. You will probably have to experiment with your technique if you want to achieve a sustained walking speed of 4 mph or faster. As always, start easy and incrementally increase the difficulty.

CHAPTER TWO

Equipment Preparation

ESSENTIAL GEAR OVERVIEW

The only absolutely essential gear for rucking is a functional backpack with some weight inside and clothing appropriate for the environmental conditions.

Backpack

Packs will be covered in more detail in subsequent chapters. To get started, any functional backpack will be fine as long as it can hold 5 to 20 lbs without ripping. You should invest in a well-designed pack as you start to go up in weight and start rucking longer distances.

Check out the chapters Selecting the Right Rucksack and Build an Inexpensive Rucking Pack for more information on packs.

Weight

You can fill your ruck with anything from military gear, weights, sandbags, and bottles of water. There are unlimited options. You are good to go as long as you have something that will fit your pack and is the proper amount of weight for you.

If I were to go rucking in the wilderness, I would fill my pack with practical gear that may be useful in that specific environment. If that gear is not heavy enough, I can add something else to make up for the weight.

When I ruck in an urban or suburban environment, I will often use weight plates and old clothing as filler. Whatever you use for weight, there is a system for properly distributing the weight in your pack. More on that in the Load Distribution chapter

Clothing

The clothing you choose must be appropriate for the weather conditions and environment you are rucking in. I live in New England, so I often wear shorts and T-shirts in the summer. In the winter, I'm usually in several layers of clothing, allowing me to stay warm and remove layers if I start to overheat or sweat too much. I will cover more on this in the Clothing and Weather Preparations chapter.

Footwear

Footwear is subject to individual preferences. Some people will prefer heavy boots that offer a lot of support and protection, and others, like me, prefer more minimalist footwear. Again, just like with clothing your footwear must be appropriate to the weather and environment you are rucking in. It is also critical. See the Footwear Selection and Foot Care chapter for more information on footwear.

SELECTING THE RIGHT RUCKSACK

Choosing a rucksack is very individualized. It will depend on your body's proportions and your personal preferences for comfort. You can purchase a rucksack, but in the next section, I will share some tips on building a rucksack with military surplus gear. Whether you use military gear or civilian gear, there are some general guidelines.

When choosing a backpack or rucksack, especially for activities like rucking, hiking, camping, or extended travel, there are several important factors to consider to ensure that you get a pack that suits your needs and is comfortable to carry. Here are some key features and aspects to look for:

Size and Capacity: The size of the backpack, often measured in liters, should be chosen based on the amount of gear you need to carry.

Fit and Comfort: The backpack should fit well on your body. Look for adjustable shoulder straps, hip belts, and chest straps. The hip belt should sit on your hips, not your waist, to distribute weight effectively.

Frame Type: Decide between an internal or external frame based on your needs. Internal frames are more common, offer better mobility, and are suitable for most hiking trips. External frames are good for heavy loads and offer better ventilation.

Material and Durability: The material should be durable and able to withstand the rigors of your activity. Nylon and polyester are common for their strength and water resistance. Check the denier rating; higher numbers usually mean tougher material.

Water Resistance: Most backpacks are not completely waterproof, having water-resistant material or a rain cover is important for keeping your gear dry.

Weight: A lighter backpack can reduce overall load, but don't sacrifice durability and comfort for the sake of weight.

Ventilation: A backpack with good back ventilation can prevent excessive sweating.

Load Adjustment Features: Features like load lifter straps, compression straps, and adjustable torso lengths can help balance and stabilize the load for a more comfortable carry.

Try on the backpack with some weight in it to get a feel for how it carries. A good fit and comfort are crucial, especially for longer trips or heavy loads.

Frame

Backpack frames serve several important functions in the design and use of backpacks, especially those used for hiking, camping, or carrying heavy loads. Here are the primary functions:

Weight Distribution: One of the most crucial functions of a backpack frame is evenly distributing the load's weight. This helps reduce strain on any part of the body, especially the shoulders and lower back. By distributing weight more evenly, the frame allows for a more comfortable carrying experience over longer periods or distances.

Stability and Balance: Frames provide structure to the backpack, which helps in maintaining balance and stability. This is particularly important when navigating uneven terrain, as it prevents the contents from shifting too much, which could throw off the wearer's balance.

Load Support: The frame supports the weight of the contents, preventing the backpack from sagging or losing shape. This is important for both the backpack's longevity and the wearer's comfort. A well-supported load is easier to carry and can reduce fatigue.

Improved Comfort: Many backpack frames are designed with ergonomics in mind. They often include features like a contoured shape that matches the curve of the wearer's back, padded areas to reduce pressure points, and channels or mesh panels to improve airflow and reduce sweat.

Attachment Points: Frames often provide structural points where additional gear can be attached. This is useful for items that are too large or awkward to fit inside the backpack's main compartment, such as sleeping pads, tents, or trekking poles.

Enhanced Load Carrying Capacity: With a frame, backpacks can typically handle heavier loads than frameless designs. This makes framed backpacks a preferred choice for activities that require carrying a lot of gear, like rucking, hiking, extended camping trips or mountaineering expeditions.

There are two main types of backpack frames: external and internal. External frames are visible from the outside and usually consist of a rigid structure to which the bag and other components are attached. Internal frames are built into the backpack and are not visible from the outside, providing a more streamlined appearance and often a closer, more body-hugging fit. Each type has its advantages and is suited to different activities and preferences.

Shoulder Straps

When evaluating the straps of a backpack or rucksack, it's important to consider several key factors to ensure comfort, durability, and effective weight distribution. Here are the primary things to look for in backpack straps:

Padding: Look for straps with adequate padding to provide comfort and cushioning, especially if you'll be carrying heavy loads. The padding should be thick enough to prevent the straps from digging into your shoulders but not so bulky that it restricts movement or causes overheating.

Width and Shape: The straps should be wide enough to distribute weight evenly across your shoulders without causing pressure points. Ergonomically shaped straps that contour to your body can enhance comfort and stability.

Adjustability: Adjustable straps allow you to customize the fit of the backpack to your body size and shape. This includes the ability to adjust the length of the shoulder straps and the position of the sternum (chest) strap and hip belt, if present.

Breathability: Ventilated or mesh straps can help reduce sweating and increase comfort, especially in warmer climates or during strenuous activities.

Sternum (Chest) Strap: This strap helps to stabilize the load and distribute weight more evenly. It should be adjustable both in length and height to ensure it sits comfortably across your chest.

Load Lifter Straps: These are located at the top of the shoulder straps and help to pull the weight of the pack closer to your body, improving balance and reducing strain on your shoulders and back.

Hip Belt Compatibility: If your backpack has a hip belt, ensure that the shoulder straps work well in conjunction with it. The hip belt should take most of the weight off your shoulders, so the straps shouldn't be overly tight once the belt is fastened.

Attachment Points: Some backpacks have additional loops or clips on the straps for attaching gear or routing hydration hoses.

Ease of Use: Straps should be easy to adjust, even when wearing gloves or with cold hands.

Reflective Elements: For added safety, especially in low-light conditions, look for straps with reflective materials.

Remember, the best way to evaluate backpack straps is to try the backpack on with some weight in it. This will give you the most accurate feel for how the straps will perform under load.

Waist Belt

When selecting a backpack or rucksack, the waist belt is crucial, especially for larger packs designed for extended trips or heavy loads. Here are the key features to look for in a waist belt:

Padding: Adequate padding in the waist belt is essential for comfort, particularly when carrying heavier loads. The padding should be thick enough to cushion your hips but not so bulky that it restricts movement.

Width and Fit: A wider waist belt can distribute weight more effectively and reduce pressure points. It should fit snugly around your hips, not your waist, to effectively transfer the load from your back and shoulders to your hips and legs.

Adjustability: Look for a waist belt that is easily adjustable, allowing you to tighten or loosen it for a custom fit. This is important for accommodating different layers of clothing and ensuring comfort throughout your journey.

Material and Durability: The material of the waist belt should be durable and able to withstand wear and tear. High-quality fabrics like nylon or polyester are commonly used. Also, check the stitching and fastenings for robustness.

Breathability: A waist belt with good ventilation or breathable materials can help reduce sweating and increase comfort, especially in warm weather or during strenuous activity.

Load Transfer: The belt should effectively transfer the pack's weight from your shoulders to your hips. This is crucial for reducing fatigue and improving balance.

Ease of Use: The belt should be easy to fasten and adjust, even when wearing gloves or with cold hands.

Compatibility with the Backpack: Ensure that the waist belt complements the backpack's overall design and doesn't interfere with other features, like side pockets or compression straps.

Sturdy Buckle: The buckle should be strong and easy to clip and unclip. It should also be reliable, so it doesn't accidentally release under the weight of the pack.

Seam Construction: Look for reinforced seams where the belt attaches to the backpack, as this area is subject to significant stress and strain.

Ergonomic Design: Some waist belts are ergonomically shaped to fit the contours of your body more naturally, which can enhance comfort and stability.

Remember, the best way to determine if a waist belt is suitable is to try on the backpack with some weight in it. This allows you to feel how the belt distributes weight and fits around your hips.

BUILD AN INEXPENSIVE RUCKSACK

What Is Needed for Rucking?

Other than appropriate clothing and footwear. You only need a backpack and something to put in the pack for weight. The pack you choose must be sturdy enough to handle your load. However, as you increase the weight, comfort becomes an important consideration. This article will focus on making a rugged, comfortable, cheap rucksack.

Rucking Weight

It's essential to keep in mind weight is relative. What is considered heavy and light depends on the size, age, gender, and fitness level of the individual. A 100-pound woman and a 250-pound man should probably not be targeting the same pack weights. Any weights mentioned in this article are just examples and rules of thumb; don't take them too seriously.

Lighter Weights

Almost any sturdy backpack will be fine if you are rucking with lighter weights, generally below 20 lbs. Start by using whatever you have, and if there are no comfort issues, stick with that until you can increase the weight.

Heavier Weights

As you increase the weight of your rucksack, weight distribution becomes an important consideration. The shoulder straps, waist belt, and frame become increasingly important in helping you to carry your pack comfortably. I've had to carry heavy packs for long distances where I couldn't properly adjust for the load, and it was miserable. I don't recommend doing it unless you have to.

Packs Designed for Rucking

Military Surplus Packs

Consider looking at military surplus packs if you want a heavy-duty pack suitable for rucking with heavier loads. You can assemble a versatile, rugged pack for around $100 to $125, especially if you are willing to shop around. I have experimented extensively with military surplus packs and found several combinations of old-style Alice packs and newer Molle gear that work well together.

Components of Rucksack

The Pack

The first component I recommend is a medium Alice pack. Medium Alice packs are cheap and plentiful. They are also light, rugged, and a good size for weight distribution. I have also experimented with large Alice packs. Large Alice packs are harder to find, more expensive, and it's more challenging to concentrate weight efficiently for rucking, but are perfectly good for rucking.

Frame

I recommend two frames: the traditional Alice Pack Frame and the Molle 1609 frame.

Alice Pack Frame

Actual Army issue Alice pack frames are getting harder to come by and more expensive. I will occasionally see them reasonably priced on sites where people sell used items. You will pay much more if you get one from an Army Surplus store. These are good to get if you can, but I don't recommend paying top dollar just to get one for rucking.

Knock-off Alice Pack Frames

Because of the availability of medium Alice packs and the lack of Army issue frames, there is a demand for third-party knock-off frames. While these knock-offs are inferior to the original frames, they are much cheaper, and I have found them to be perfectly adequate for rucking. Would I want to use them in a tactical combat situation? No, but I have never had an issue with knock-off frames for walking around with a weighted pack. Your experience might vary.

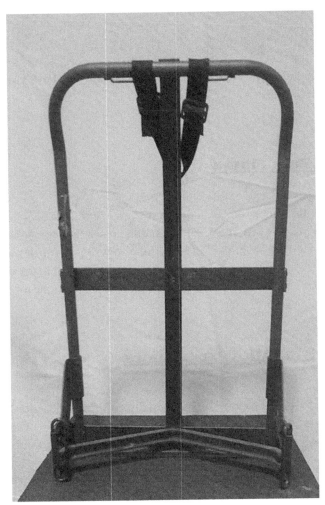

Alice Pack Frame

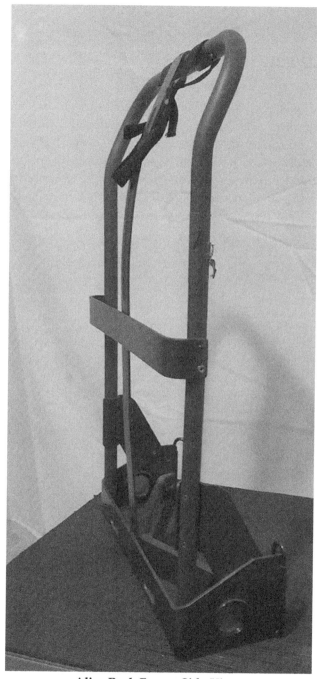

Alice Pack Frame Side View

1609 Open Molle Frame

The 1609 Open Molle Frame has become my go-to frame for the medium Alice pack. They are light and comfortable. I hesitate to use these if you ruck with weights greater than 60 lbs, but very few people will ruck with that much weight outside the military. Also, if you are going to use a 1609 frame with an Alice waist belt, you will have to do a small modification. I'll discuss that more later on.

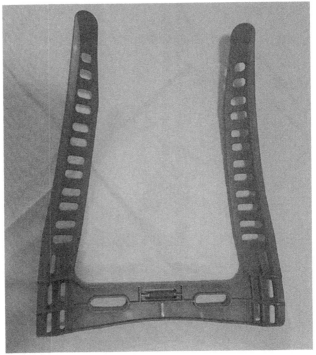

Molle 1609 Frame

Shoulder Straps

Alice Pack Shoulder Straps

Like Army-issue Alice frames, Army-issue Alice shoulder straps are getting hard to find. In my opinion, Army-issue Alice shoulder straps are not ideal for rucking, especially with heavy loads. So I don't recommend them. The cheap knock-offs that are available should be avoided at all costs. If you get a pack with cheap knock-offs included, I recommend throwing them away.

There are some more expensive Alice-compatible, third-party straps that I do like for rucking, but they will add to the overall costs. One third-party maker of Alice pack-compatible straps I've had good luck with is Fire Force. I'm sure there are other brands out there, but I recommend these if you are willing to spend a few extra dollars.

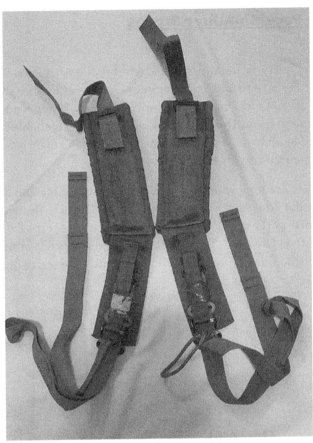
Army Issue Alice Pack Straps

Molle Shoulder Straps

If you are trying to save every dollar possible. I recommend going with Molle-style shoulder straps. They are comfortable, cheap, and can be used with Alice and Molle frames. In my experience, these straps do a great job of distributing weight on your shoulders. The downside with Molle straps is that you cannot match the color to your Alice pack. Personally, I don't care about that, but some people might.

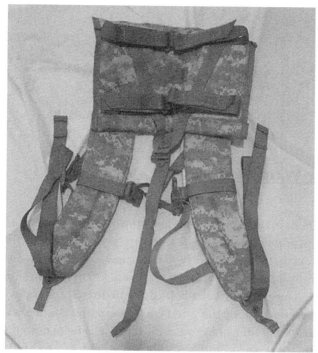

Molle Rucking Shoulder Straps

Waist Belts

Alice Pack Waist Belts

Again, Army-issue Alice pack waist belts are getting harder to find, but I have found them to be adequate for rucking. If you go with a third-party Alice-compatible waist belt, again, I've found the Fire Force brand to be excellent. Alice pack waist belts can obviously be used with Alice frames. If you want to use them with Molle 1609 frames, you must modify the frame slightly. I will discuss this later on.

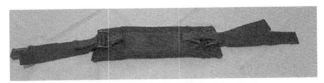
Army Issue Alice Pack Waist Belt

Molle Waist Belts

There are two Molle waist belt styles: one for larger packs and another for medium-sized packs. Many people swear by the belt for large packs. I have not had good experiences with them. To be fair, I believe my problems were directly related to my being short, but I found the large Molle waist belts dug into my glutes and were extremely uncomfortable, and I was never able to find a way around this. Because of this, I recommend using Molle belts designed for medium-sized packs. Both styles of Molle belts can be used with Alice pack frames and the Molle 1609 frames.

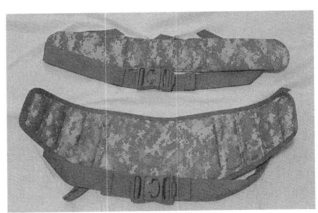
Large and Medium Molle Waist Belts

Weight for the Pack

You can literally use anything that will fit into your bag for weight. Ideally, it's best to distribute the weight as close to your body as possible, and the heaviest weight should be up near your shoulders.

Among other things, I've used sandbags, weight plates, dumbbells, and weight vests. You will probably have to experiment with packing and distributing the weight, but your goal is to pack the weight close to your body and up near your shoulders. Also, pack it tightly enough so the weight will not be shifting around. I use cloth and other lightweight materials as filler when needed.

Recommended Configurations for Mixing and Matching Items

The Hellcat Alice/Molle Hybrid Pack

A popular Alice pack mod is called the Hellcat Mod among bushcraft community members. For rucking, I recommend a slightly modified version of this configuration. You won't need the Molle sleep system carrier. However, if you choose to include it, that's fine.

This configuration includes a medium Alice pack, an Alice frame, Molle shoulder straps, and a Molle waist belt. Again, I recommend the Molle waist belt for medium packs, but many people use the belt for large packs.

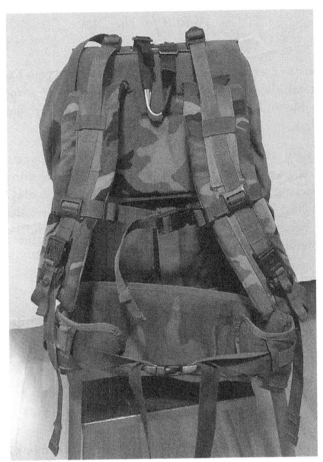

Hellcat Configuration

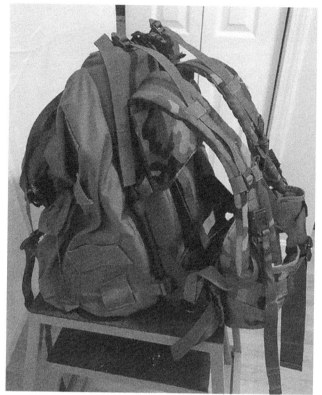

Hellcat Configuration Side View

Here is a link to instructions on how to put the pack together - here!

Modified Hellcat Pack using an Alice Belt

This is my go-to configuration for rucking with heavy loads. It is the same as the original Hellcat modification, except the Molle waist belt is replaced with an Alice pack-compatible waist belt. Fire Force manufactures the one I use.

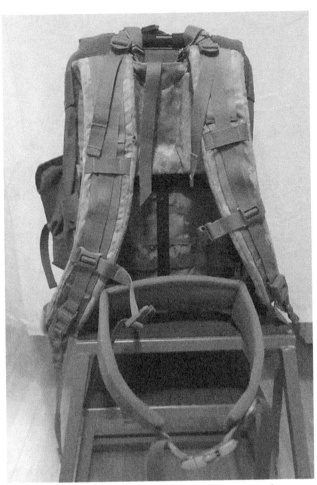

Hellcat Configuration with an Alice Belt

Modified Hellcat Pack using the Molle 1609 Frame

This is a great configuration if you also want to use your pack as a day pack. It consists of a medium Alice pack, a 1609 frame, Molle Straps, and either a Mollie or an Alice waist belt. Again, I recommend the medium Mollie waist belt. You must modify the frame slightly if you use an Alice waist belt. More on that later.

If I had to choose only one configuration, it would be this one. This configuration is the most inexpensive and can double as an excellent hiking pack.

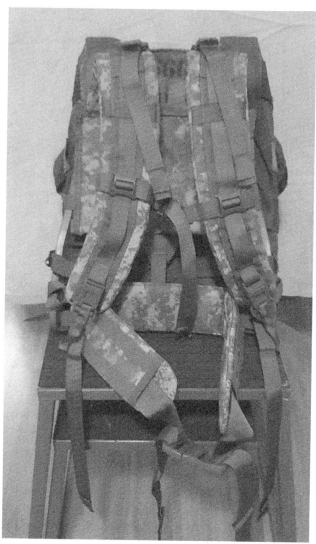

Hellcat Configuration with a 1609 Frame

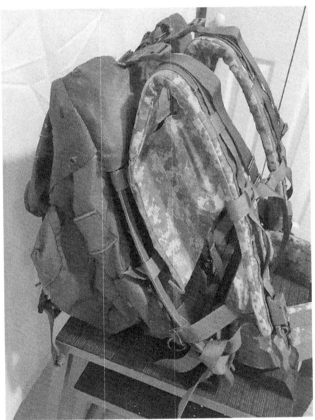

Hellcat Configuration with a 1609 Frame Side View

Traditional Alice Pack Configuration

Some people use Alice packs with Alice frames, shoulder straps, and waist belt. If you want to go with this configuration, replace standard-issue Alice straps with Fire Force Alice-compatible shoulder straps and the waist belt as well.

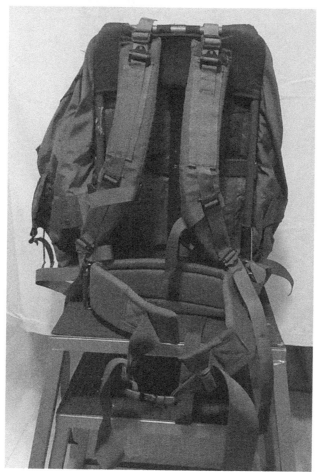

Traditional Alice pack configuration using Fire Force belt and straps

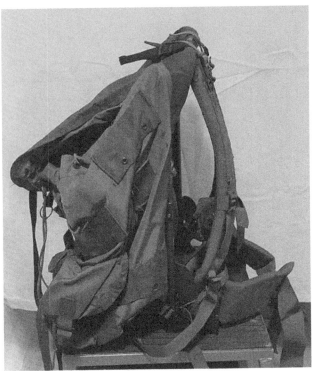

Traditional Alice pack configuration using Fire Force belt and straps

Bare-bones Configuration

This configuration consists of an Alice pack frame and any shoulder strap and belt combo you prefer, but no pack. You will also need to buy an Alice pack frame shelf. With this configuration, the weight is strapped or secured directly to the Alice pack frame on top of the Alice pack shelf at the bottom of the frame. The weights are usually metal plates of some kind.

Personally, I haven't used this setup. Clearly, this is a single-purpose setup for rucking. If you also want to use your ruck as a general-purpose backpack, then this probably is not the best configuration.

Modifying the 1609 Frame for Alice Compatible Belts

If you use an Alice-compatible belt with a 1609 frame, you will have to cut out two small sections in the bottom corners of the frame. I easily accomplished this with a handheld hacksaw.

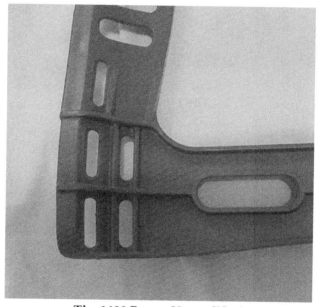

The 1609 Frame Unmodified

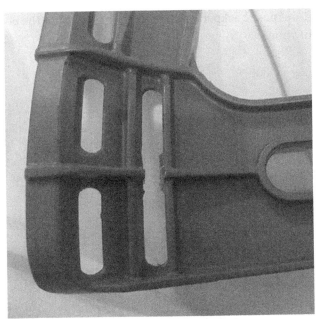

The 1609 Frame Modified

Final Thoughts

As a general rule of thumb, the more weight you plan to carry, the more you should consider using an Alice pack frame. You probably could go up to 60 or so pounds with the Molle frame, but it's up to you. If you want to have a versatile Alice pack system, consider getting a medium Molle belt, Molle straps, Molle frame, and an Alice pack frame. Depending on the load, you can change the frame as needed.

Places to Shop for the Equipment

I've used the following resources to buy my equipment. Take your time and bargain hunt.

Amazon.com: Amazon is always a good place to start. I have found some great deals there, but there is also a lot of overpriced stuff.

Ebay.com: I have found a lot of good deals on gear there. Prices will vary considerably.

Facebook Marketplace: I regularly see full Alice packs with frames, straps, and belts for sale here at good prices.

Military Surplus Stores: The prices and available equipment vary widely if you use Military Surplus stores. Do not assume that you are going to get a good deal.

Fireforceusa.com: Good after-market Alice-compatible Belts and Straps.

CLOTHING AND WEATHER PREPARATION

Dressing appropriately for rucking is crucial for both comfort and safety. What you wear will depend on the weather and the environment in which you are operating. Temperature, humidity, and exposure to the sun (known as solar load) will determine specifically what you should wear. Below are some general guidelines.

Layered Clothing

Wear multiple layers of clothing. This allows you to adjust your body temperature easily as you warm up or cool down. Typically, three layers are recommended. You will need to adjust based on the conditions. In hot weather, you may not need anything but a thin base layer. In general, you can use layers to adjust to your needs. You can strip off or put on these layers as needed to remain comfortable.

Base Layer: This should be moisture-wicking to keep sweat away from your skin. Materials like merino wool or synthetic fibers work well.

Insulation Layer: This layer retains body heat to protect you from the cold. Fleece jackets or down vests are good choices.

Outer Layer: A waterproof and windproof jacket is essential, especially in unpredictable weather conditions.

Pants

Choose rucking pants made from durable, quick-drying fabrics like nylon or spandex. Avoid cotton as it takes a long time to dry and doesn't provide good insulation when wet. Wool pants are also a good option in cold weather.

Footwear

Footwear needs to fit your foot properly. You may need to go up in size to accommodate thick socks in colder environments. Shoes that are too big can cause problems by allowing your foot to slide around, causing instability on hills and rocking terrain. Shoes that are too small will cause blisters and a painful situation called toe-jamming when your toes push up against the front of your shoes.

In warmer environments, to prevent blisters, you want boots or shoes that breathe, preventing sweat from accumulating and keeping your feet as dry as possible.

You will need boots that keep your feet warm and dry in colder weather. They will also need to breathe; otherwise, you run the risk of your sweat freezing and frostbite.

In general, for short rucks, you will not have to worry too much about your footwear unless you are in a very extreme environment. For longer rucks, you must have shoes that will protect your feet from the weather and the environment, particularly if you are rucking in the wilderness.

Socks

Opt for moisture-wicking and breathable rucking socks. Wool or synthetic blends are preferable over cotton. Cotton is a really bad choice for socks. It retains sweat and water and dries slowly. Once cotton socks are wet, they will likely cause blisters.

Personally, I have yet to find anything better than wool. I only wear wool socks even when it's very hot. Here's why.

- Wool breathes, keeping one's feet cool when it's hot and dry when it's cold.

- Wool prevents blisters. If my shoes fit correctly, I never get blisters with wool socks.

- Wool drys easily because it doesn't retain water very well.

- Wool is antimicrobial and will not stink as much from perspiration and sweat.

Carrying extra socks never hurts when rucking long distances, particularly in cold, wet weather.

Hat and Gloves

Depending on the weather, a hat can protect you from the sun or keep you warm in cold conditions. Gloves are essential in colder weather.

Rain Gear: Always pack lightweight rain gear, even if the weather forecast is clear. Weather in mountainous areas can be unpredictable.

Sun Protection: Wear a hat with a brim. Wear sunglasses and apply sunscreen to exposed skin.

Bring an Extra Layer Just In Case

I always recommend bringing an extra layer in case you are forced to stop. When you are rucking, you will be burning calories that will help keep you warm. If you must stop for an extended period of time, you will likely need the extra layer to keep you warm until you can move out.

Adjust as the Weather and Environment Dictate

The specific gear you need may vary depending on the length of your ruck, the weather, and the terrain. Always check the weather forecast and trail conditions before heading out, and adjust your clothing and gear accordingly.

FOOTWEAR SELECTION AND FOOT CARE

Choosing the right footwear for rucking is crucial for comfort and safety, especially for longer rucks. Here are some key factors to consider.

Terrain

The terrain type will determine the footwear you need.

Flat or Gentle Trails: Light-rucking shoes or sneakers are suitable.

Rugged or Mountainous Terrain: rucking boots with good ankle support and tough soles are recommended.

Fit and Comfort

Size: Ensure there's a thumb's width of space in front of your toes. This provides room for your feet to swell and prevents your toes from hitting the front of the boot on downhill treks.

Width: The shoes should be snug but not tight, with enough room to wiggle your toes.

Try Before You Buy: Always try on rucking footwear with the socks you plan to ruck in.

Material

Leather: Durable and offers great support and protection but can be heavy and less breathable.

Synthetic Materials: Lighter and more breathable but may not offer as much durability and protection.

Waterproofing

Waterproof shoes are essential if you're rucking in wet conditions. However, they can be less breathable in hot, dry conditions. This may not be as important for short rucks, but as your distances increase, you want to prevent your feet from being wet for an extended period.

Sole and Grip: Look for sturdy soles with deep lugs for good traction, especially if you're rucking on slippery or uneven surfaces.

Weight: Lighter shoes are less tiring over long distances but may offer less support and protection.

Durability: Consider how often you ruck and in what conditions. More durable materials may be heavier but can better withstand rough terrain.

Breaking In: It is important to break in new rucking footwear with short walks before going on longer rucks to prevent blisters and discomfort.

Remember, the best rucking footwear is the one that fits you well and suits the specific conditions of your ruck. Investing in quality footwear is worth ensuring your rucking experience is enjoyable and safe.

CHAPTER THREE

Technique and Load Distribution

LOAD DISTRIBUTION

Load distribution is very important. If the weight is not distributed properly, your ruck will slow you down, be uncomfortable, and cause needless wear and tear on your back and joints.

Two things to remember: pack the weight close and then pack it up. What do I mean by that?

Pack the Weight Close

You want to pack the heaviest part of the load so it sits in the pack up next to your body. If you pack it so the weight is the outer part of the pack, it will act as a counterbalance to moving forward. In other words, it will pull you back and make it much harder to move forward.

Pack the Weight Up

Ideally, you want to pack the weight so it sits up next to your shoulders. This will move your center of gravity higher, making it easier to disrupt your balance and fall forward as you lean into your stride.

The lower your weight, the lower your center of gravity will be. This will make you more stable and prevent you from falling forward.

Start with an Empty Pack

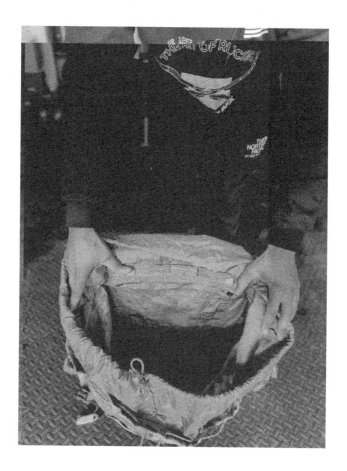

Place Lighter Items In the Bottom

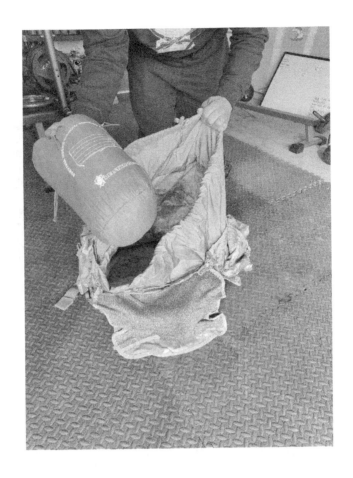

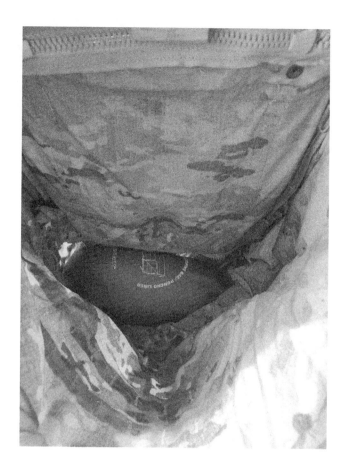

Place the Heavier Items on the Top Toward the Back

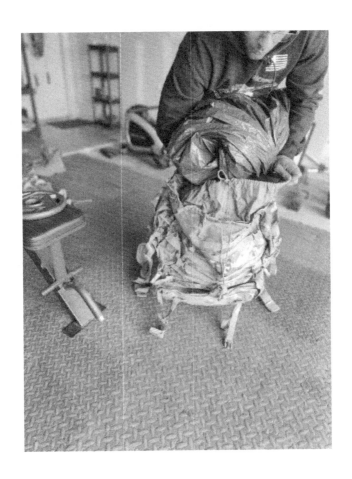

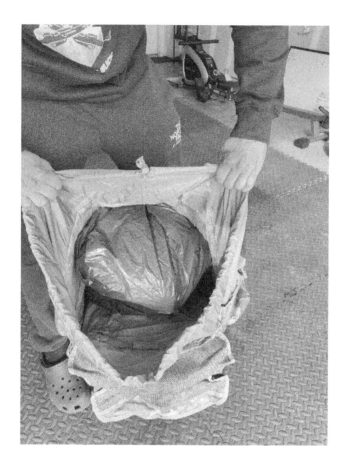

<u>Finish by Filling with Light Weight Material in the Front</u>

Take some old crumpled clothes, crumpled paper, or anything else that can be used as lightweight padding, and place them in front of the heavy items to prevent them from moving around. **You do not want to give the items in your pack room to shift around.**

TECHNIQUE

Technique is one of the most overlooked elements in walking and running. While walking and running are not exactly the same biomechanically, they are similar enough that most people exhibit the same flaws when walking and running. Generally, rucking is most similar to walking so everything I discuss here will apply equally to walking, running and rucking.

Speed can be determined by a simple formula - **Stride Length x Cadence.**

The Relationship Between Stride Length and Speed

As you increase your speed, your stride length will naturally increase. However, the opposite is not true. Increasing your stride length will not increase your speed. This is a subtle but important point. Stride length is determined by speed, but speed is not determined by stride length.

Why is this? When you increase your stride length without increasing your cadence, you will be overstriding (see below), and your leg will act as a break, slowing you down.

The Relationship Between Cadence and Speed

Increasing your cadence, which is the number of steps you take per minute, will increase your speed. That is assuming you do not decrease your stride length. Normally, as you increase your cadence, your stride length will either stay the same or increase to accommodate the faster speed at which you are moving.

Overstriding: The Most Common Technical Error

Contrary to popular belief, walking, running, and rucking is not a series of pushes forward. In other words, you do not push yourself forward. You move forward by falling while supported with one leg and landing on the other. In other words, you move forward via a series of falls.

The leg you fall onto must touch the ground as close to your center of gravity as possible. The further you land out in front of your body, the more your leg will act as a break.

Unfortunately, all the energy you lose from going forward has to go somewhere. As it turns out, It goes up into your leg, causing wear and tear on your joints and bones. If you have sore knees, hips, or ankles, that is a good sign you are overstriding. Another common sign of overstriding is shin splints.

Good Technique vs. Overstriding

Here are two examples of **Michael Noexcuse** rucking. One shows good technique, and the other shows overstriding.

Good Technique

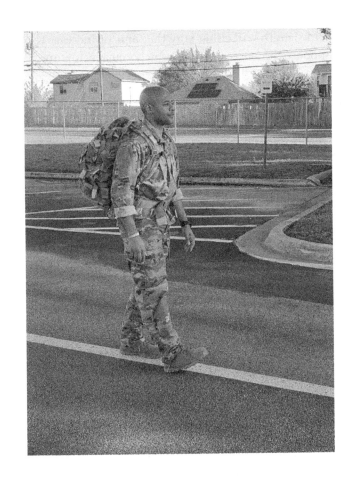

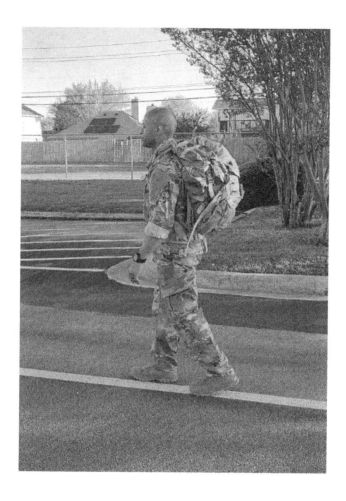

In the pictures above, Michael demonstrates good technique by placing his foot near his center of gravity.

Bad Technique

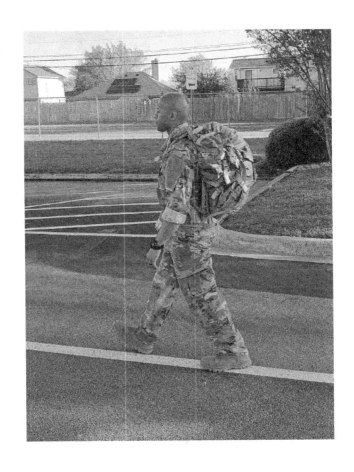

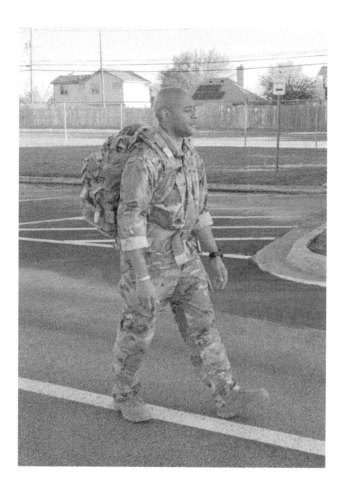

In these pictures, Michael is landing way out in front of his center of gravity, breaking a little with each step, which causes his cadence to drop.

Rucking on Flat Ground

When rucking on flat ground, focus on landing as close to your center of gravity as possible. To increase your speed, lean forward and increase your cadence. Your stride length will naturally increase as needed. If you are landing close to your center of gravity, then your stride length should be where it needs to be.

Rucking Downhill

If you overstride while going downhill, the forces will be magnified, and you will be doing even more damage to your joints and bones. When going downhill, do not lean into your stride, collapse your supporting leg, and catch yourself on your other leg. It's like going down a staircase without the stairs.

Rucking Uphill

When going uphill, overstriding is not as big of an issue. Most people naturally shorten their stride because overstriding will become very tiring. When going uphill, it's important to use short, quick strides. Again, it's like walking up a staircase without the stairs.

CHAPTER FOUR

Physical Training

TYPES OF EXERCISE

I categorize fitness into two broad categories: physiological and neurological. Physiological fitness is what most people think about when they start an exercise program. It covers endurance (cardio), muscular endurance, stamina, strength and power. Other people may categorize things differently, and that's fine, but I've been involved in the fitness world for nearly 50 years as of this writing, and this is what works for me.

Physiological

Endurance

Endurance is about low to moderately intense exercise for a long period of time. Forms of endurance training include, but are not limited to, walking, hiking, rucking, running, biking, and rowing.

The primary benefit of endurance exercise is improving cardiovascular fitness and metabolism by stimulating the production of mitochondria, which use oxygen and glycogen to produce energy for the body. The more mitochondria you have, the more efficiently you can produce energy for your body.

Strength

Strength is about increasing the force of muscular contractions and is the basis of all physical activity. Every movement requires some element of strength. Depending on the movement, it may not be a lot of strength, but the more athletic the movements, the more strength becomes a limiting factor.

Power

Muscular power refers to the ability of a muscle or group of muscles to produce the maximum amount of force in the shortest possible time. It combines both strength and speed. In other words, it's the rate at which work is done or energy is transferred. Muscular power is crucial for activities that require quick bursts of effort, such as jumping, sprinting, or throwing. It is often assessed by measuring the performance in exercises like vertical jumps or short sprints. Training for muscular power typically involves plyometric exercises or lifting weights at a faster velocity.

Stamina

In the context of physical training, stamina refers to the ability of an individual to sustain prolonged physical or mental effort without experiencing undue fatigue. It is often used interchangeably with "endurance," though stamina can sometimes emphasize the mental aspect of pushing through fatigue in addition to the physical.

Stamina encompasses:

Cardiovascular Stamina: Relates to the heart and lungs' ability to deliver oxygen to the working muscles during prolonged physical activity. It's crucial for activities like running, cycling, and swimming over extended distances.

Muscular Stamina: This refers to a muscle's or group of muscles' ability to perform repeated contractions over a period without fatigue. It's essential for activities that require sustained muscle activity, such as holding a plank position or doing multiple repetitions of an exercise.

Mental Stamina: While physical training primarily focuses on the body, the mind plays a significant role in pushing through barriers, maintaining focus, and staying motivated during extended periods of exertion.

Improving stamina is a common goal in physical training, and it can be achieved through various exercises and training regimens, including aerobic activities, interval training, and resistance training. Enhanced stamina allows individuals to perform activities for longer durations and at higher intensities without quickly succumbing to fatigue.

Neurological

Joint Mobility

Joint mobility is more commonly known as flexibility. Contrary to popular belief, flexibility has little to do with the tissues of the muscles and tendons. Your brain controls flexibility via something called "neurological inhibition." This is a very complicated subject, but your brain is trying to protect you from doing things that might cause injury and will tell the muscles to tighten if it perceives that you might get injured.

Joint mobility is the range of uninhibited movement around a joint or a series of joints. It encompasses the ability of a joint to move freely and smoothly through its full range of motion (ROM). Joint mobility is influenced by several factors, including the shape and structure of the bones, the condition of the ligaments and tendons surrounding the joint, the elasticity of the muscles, and the presence or absence of any obstructions or abnormalities within the joint.

Good joint mobility can contribute to improved athletic performance, reduced risk of injury, and better overall function in daily activities. Conversely, restricted mobility can lead to discomfort, pain, or a decreased ability to perform certain movements or tasks. Regular stretching, mobility exercises, and maintaining an active lifestyle can help preserve and enhance joint mobility.

Balance

Regarding human movement, balance refers to the ability to maintain the body's center of mass over its base of support. It involves the coordination of various sensory inputs (from the eyes, ears, and proprioceptors in the muscles and joints) and motor responses to achieve and maintain a stable position or to control the body's position during movement.

There are several components to balance:

Static Balance: The ability to maintain stability when standing still, without moving.

Dynamic Balance: The ability to remain balanced in motion or switching between different positions.

Reactive Balance: The ability to recover stability after an unexpected disturbance, such as a push or trip.

Anticipatory Balance: The ability to proactively stabilize the body in preparation for a voluntary movement, like lifting a leg or reaching out.

Balance is crucial for everyday activities and is a fundamental skill in many sports and physical activities. It can be improved through specific exercises and training, and its importance increases with age as balance tends to decline, increasing the risk of falls and related injuries.

Skill

Skill is the ability to perform a specific task or movement with precision, efficiency, and coordination. It involves the integration of sensory inputs (such as vision and proprioception) with motor functions to produce a desired outcome. Skills can be simple, like picking up an object, or complex, like executing a gymnastics routine or playing a musical instrument.

Key components of skill in human movement include:

Coordination: The harmonious functioning of muscles or groups of muscles in executing complex movements.

Precision: The ability to execute a movement accurately and consistently.

Adaptability: The capacity to adjust one's movements based on changing conditions or environments.

Timing: Synchronizing movements in relation to external factors, such as hitting a ball at the right moment.

Efficiency: Performing a movement with minimal wasted effort or energy.

Fluency: The smoothness and flow of a movement without unnecessary interruptions or hesitations.

Skills can be innate to some extent, but they are primarily developed and refined through practice, training, and experience. The process of skill acquisition often involves progressing from clumsy, conscious efforts to more fluid, automatic actions as one becomes more proficient.

EXERCISE GUIDELINES

The Goal is Improved Health

For the purpose of this book, the goal is to get healthy, not to pursue your athletic potential, which, if done incorrectly, can negatively affect your health.

Everyone has a unique combination of strengths and weaknesses that determine how fit they are, what they should focus on, and what their potential is. I'm sure there are people reading this who are active and fit and others who are on the other end of the fitness spectrum. So, I can't prescribe a one-size-fits-all program for everyone, but I'll give you some guidelines.

Check Your Ego the Door

You must put your ego aside and accept your fitness level as it is. Otherwise, you are setting yourself up for injury. A big part of success is dealing with the reality of your circumstances. Denial is the path to failure. That is true of fitness, and it is true of dealing with every other problem in life.

Focus on Your Weaknesses

Most people love to work on their strengths because it feeds their egos. To seek a healthy balance, focus on what you are NOT good at.

Don't Neglect Your Strengths

While you should focus on your weaknesses, don't completely neglect your strengths, or you may find them becoming your weaknesses.

Seek to Establish a Balanced Program

The healthiest exercise programs are balanced programs. Ideally, you will become reasonably comfortable with all elements of fitness. Unfortunately, it's much harder than it sounds, but it's best to put enough variety in your program to touch on most fitness elements.

Don't Drive Yourself Crazy Seeking Perfect Exercise Program

Don't let perfection become the enemy of the good. It is not reasonable to try to develop the perfect exercise program. I don't believe there is any such thing. Even top athletes have room for improvement. The important thing is to do something; the next most important thing is to add variety. Don't become obsessed with too many goals and variables.

Improve Gradually and then Maintain

Your goal is to gradually improve your physical capacity. Once you are happy with your fitness level, the goal is to maintain it. Alternatively, you can maintain what you have been working on and refocus on your weaknesses. The key word here is "gradually." Set reasonable, achievable goals.

Consistency

It is far better to exercise for a few minutes every day than to exercise for a lot of time occasionally. Make some form of exercise part of your daily routine. If you start running and need to rest, go for a walk or do some stretching, but do something.

Pain vs Discomfort

Exercise should be uncomfortable, especially when you are getting started. It is generally okay to push through mild discomfort. Conversely, pain indicates that you are about to injure yourself, have already injured yourself, or are exacerbating a pre-existing injury. Do not push through pain!

BASIC CONDITIONING WITH A RUCKSACK

Ruck-ups

Starting Position: Lie on your back with your knees bent and feet flat on the ground. Hold your rucksack at your chest with both hands. Ensure you use a weight appropriate for you and this exercise.

Engage Core: Tighten your abdominal muscles. This will be important for stability throughout the exercise.

Initiate Sit-Up: Begin by lifting your upper body off the ground, using your core muscles, not momentum. Keep the weight close to your chest as you sit up.

Sitting Position: Continue the sit-up until your torso is vertical or nearly vertical.

Overhead Press: Once you are in the upright sitting position, press the weight overhead. Extend your arms fully, but avoid locking your elbows. Keep your core engaged to maintain balance and control.

Lower the Weight: Bring the weight back down to your chest in a controlled manner.

Return to Start: Slowly lower your upper body back to the ground to return to the starting position.

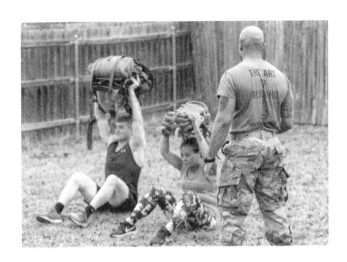

Ruck Squats

Performing squats while wearing a rucksack adds extra weight, changing the dynamics of the exercise.

Rucksack Position: Wear the rucksack on your back with an appropriate weight for this exercise. It should be snug but comfortable, with the weight evenly distributed.

Starting Stance: Stand with your feet shoulder-width apart or slightly wider. Your toes can be pointed slightly outward.

Posture: Keep your back straight, chest up, and look forward. This helps maintain a neutral spine.

Engage Core: Tighten your core muscles for stability.

Initiate the Squat: Shift your hips back and bend your knees as if sitting back into a chair.

Depth: Aim to lower yourself until your thighs are at least parallel to the ground. Ensure your knees don't go too far beyond your toes and stay aligned with your feet.

Weight Distribution: Keep your weight primarily in your heels and midfoot – you should be able to wiggle your toes.

Arms Position: Extend your arms out in front of you for balance, if needed.

Rising Up: Push through your heels to return to the starting position. Keep your core engaged and back straight throughout the movement.

Breathing: Inhale on the way down, exhale as you push back up.

Repetitions: Perform the desired number of repetitions, maintaining form throughout.

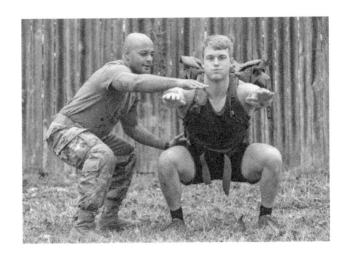

Ruck Flutter-kicks

Performing flutter kicks while holding a rucksack over your body involves core stabilization and upper-body strength.

Rucksack Preparation: Choose a rucksack with a manageable weight. Lie on your back and hold the rucksack directly above your chest with both hands. Your arms should be straight.

Positioning: Lie flat on your back on a mat. Keep your legs extended and arms straight, holding the rucksack above your chest.

Engage Core: Tighten your abdominal muscles and press your lower back into the mat for stability.

Leg Movement: Lift your heels about 6 inches off the ground. Begin to alternately kick your legs up and down in a small, controlled flutter motion.

Rucksack Stability: Keep the rucksack steady above your chest throughout the exercise. This requires upper body strength and stability.

Breathing: Breathe steadily and rhythmically throughout the exercise. Avoid holding your breath.

Completion: To finish, stop the leg movements, lower your legs to the mat, and carefully lower the rucksack to your chest before sitting up.

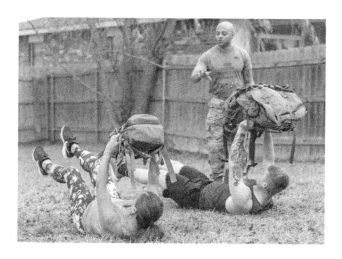

Ruck Overhead Lunges

Remember, the overhead component of this exercise increases its intensity and difficulty, especially for balance and stability. It's crucial to start with a lighter weight and focus on maintaining proper form throughout the movement.

Rucksack Preparation: Select a rucksack with a challenging but manageable weight. Secure it tightly to ensure the weight is evenly distributed.

Starting Position: Stand upright with your feet shoulder-width apart. Hold the rucksack overhead with both hands, arms fully extended. Ensure your grip is firm and your wrists are straight.

Engage Core and Shoulders: Tighten your core muscles for stability. Engage your shoulder and arm muscles to keep the rucksack steady above your head throughout the exercise.

Lunge Forward: Step forward with one leg, lowering your hips until both knees are bent at about a 90-degree angle. The front knee should be directly above your ankle, not pushed out too far. The rear knee should hover just above the ground.

Maintain Posture: Keep your upper body straight and avoid leaning forward. The rucksack should remain directly above your head, not drifting forward or backward.

Push Back Up: Push through the heel of your front foot to return to the starting position.

Alternate Legs: Repeat the movement with the opposite leg, continuing to alternate legs for the desired number of repetitions.

Breathing: Inhale as you lower into the lunge, and exhale as you push back to the starting position.

Controlled Movements: Perform the lunges in a slow and controlled manner to maintain balance and ensure proper form.

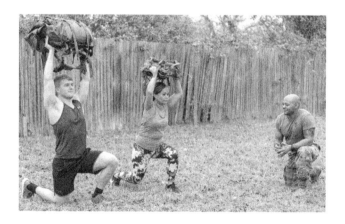

Ruck Push-ups

To perform a proper ruck push-up, follow these steps:

Done Your Rucksack: Put on your rucksack with whatever weight is appropriate for you to do this exercise.

Start Position: Begin in a plank position. Your hands should be shoulder-width apart, directly under your shoulders. Keep your feet together or slightly apart for stability. Your body should form a straight line from your head to your heels.

Engage Core: Tighten your core muscles to keep your body straight and rigid throughout the exercise.

Elbow Position: As you lower down, keep your elbows at about a 45-degree angle to your body. Avoid flaring them out too wide.

Lowering Down: Inhale as you slowly lower your body towards the ground by bending your elbows. Keep your body straight and rigid. Aim to lower yourself until your chest or chin nearly touches the floor.

Pushing Up: Exhale as you push yourself back up to the starting position by straightening your arms. Keep your core engaged and your body straight.

Repetition: Repeat the movement for your desired number of repetitions.

Remember, the focus is on maintaining proper form to maximize the effectiveness of the exercise and minimize the risk of injury.

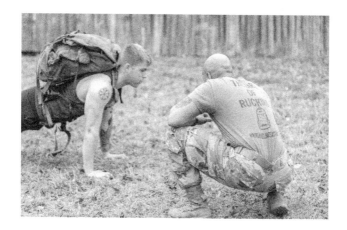

CHAPTER FIVE

Nutrition and Hydration

MACRONUTRIENTS

Warning! If you have specific dietary needs or conditions that affect your ability to eat particular types of food, consult a nutritionist before implementing my recommendations.

Diet is a big topic with a lot to cover. While I do not believe that there is a "best" diet for all people, I do believe there are general guidelines that apply to most people.

If you want a specific diet, I recommend the **Mediterranean Diet**, which is consistently ranked as one of the healthiest diets. It is not a perfect diet, but it greatly improves what most people eat in the United States.

I do not recommend extreme diets in the long term. Vegetarian, Vegan, Paleo, Keto, and similar diets may give you great results in the short term, but in the long term, these diets can result in nutritional deficiencies and metabolic problems. Of course, some people thrive on these diets, but most people will not be able to sustain these diets and remain healthy.

Ultimately, diet is personal. There will always be an element of trial and error in figuring out your individual dietary needs. Still, if you focus on the quality of your foods and finding the right balance of macronutrients, you will likely find what works for you.

Macronutrients - Proteins, Fats, and Carbohydrates

These are the Acceptable Macronutrient Distribution Ranges (AMDR) set by the Institute of Medicine of The National Academies, which provide a recommended percentage of total daily calories that should come from each macronutrient:

Carbohydrates: 45-65% of total daily calories

Proteins: 10-35% of total daily calories

Fats: 20-35% of total daily calories

For the Mediterranean Diet, the macronutrient distribution is more like this.

Carbohydrates: Around 40-50% of total daily calories. The emphasis is on complex carbs from fruits, vegetables, legumes, and whole grains.

Proteins: Around 15-20% of total daily calories. The protein mainly comes from plant sources, fish, and seafood, with poultry, eggs, cheese, and yogurt consumed less frequently and red meat more infrequently.

Fats: Approximately 30-40% of total daily calories. The fats in a Mediterranean diet are primarily unsaturated, coming from olive oil, nuts, seeds, and fatty fish.

What I Want You to Do

CARBOHYDRATES

Warning! If you have specific dietary needs or conditions that affect your ability to eat particular types of food, consult a nutritionist before implementing my recommendations.

Fruits and vegetables are the cornerstone of any healthy diet. Most people in the United States simply don't eat enough of them. You need to eat a large variety and quantity of fruits and vegetables. They tend to be low in calories and very nutrient-dense.

Grains, however, are high in calories and not very nutrient-dense. You should minimize your intake of grains. When you do eat grains, you choose unprocessed whole grains.

Glycemic Index

The glycemic index (GI) is a system that ranks foods on a scale from 1 to 100 based on their effect on blood sugar levels. Carbohydrates with a high glycemic index are digested quickly and cause a more immediate spike in your blood sugar level (i.e., glucose level). These foods include white bread, most white rices, cornflakes, and sugary drinks.

Conversely, foods with a low glycemic index are digested more slowly, causing a lower and slower rise in blood sugar levels. These include whole oats, most fruits, legumes, and non-starchy vegetables.

You should emphasize carbohydrates on the lower end of the

glycemic index.

Here is why we should avoid those on the higher end of the glycemic index.

Blood sugar spikes and crashes: High-GI foods cause rapid spikes in blood sugar, followed by sharp drops. These drops can lead to feelings of hunger, which can cause overeating and contribute to weight gain. Over time, these repeated blood sugar spikes and crashes can lead to insulin resistance, a precursor to type 2 diabetes.

Increased risk of type 2 diabetes and heart disease: Numerous studies have found that a diet high in high-GI foods can increase the risk of type 2 diabetes and heart disease. This is likely due to their impact on blood sugar levels and insulin and their potential to increase inflammation in the body.

Weight gain and obesity: High-GI foods can contribute to weight gain and obesity. They are often less satisfying than low-GI foods, leading to increased hunger and overeating. Additionally, the rapid rise and fall in blood sugar can lead to cravings for more high-GI foods.

Lack of nutrients: Many high-GI foods are also highly processed and low in fiber, vitamins, and other important nutrients. This means that while they may provide quick energy, they don't offer much in the way of long-term nutrition.

Examples:

High-GI foods (70 or higher): white rice, white bread, pretzels, white bagels, white baked potatoes, crackers, and sugar-sweetened beverages.

Medium-GI foods (56-69): bananas, grapes, spaghetti, ice cream, raisins, corn on the cob.

Low-GI foods (55 or less): oatmeal, peanuts, peas, carrots, kidney beans, hummus, skim milk, and most fruits (except those listed above and watermelon)

Eat Organic

Try to eat organic fruits and vegetables. The reason for this has nothing to do with nutrition. There is no significant nutritional difference between organic and non-organic fruits and vegetables.

Pesticides and other chemicals used on non-organic fruits and vegetables are **Endocrine Disrupting Compounds (EDCs)**. These EDCs are estrogenic, meaning they have Estrogenic properties behaving like estrogen. They mess with our Endocrine systems and alter our hormone balances. EDCs are causing quickly increasing rates of infertility in men and women and low testosterone levels in men.

If you can't get or afford organic food, please thoroughly wash your fruits and vegetables before eating them.

Nitrates and Nitric Oxide (NO)

Many health problems can be traced back to low Nitric Oxide (NO) levels. Nitrous Oxide is essential for good health. Eating fruits and vegetables high in Nitrates is important to support the ability to produce NO in adequate amounts.

Carbohydrates that Support Nitric Oxide Production

Here is a short list of fruits and vegetables high in nitrates. Eat these fruits and vegetables and add them to your diet daily.

Beetroot: Known for its exceptionally high nitrate content. Beets are often juiced or used in smoothies to provide a concentrated source of nitrates.

Spinach: Another very high source of nitrates.

Arugula (rocket): This peppery green has one of the highest nitrate contents of any vegetable.

Celery: Contains a significant amount of nitrates.

Lettuce: Red and green leaf lettuce, especially, contain high levels of nitrates.

Carrots: They're rich in nitrates as well as other nutrients.

Radishes: These root vegetables have a high nitrate content.

Collard Greens: Like other leafy green vegetables, collards are rich in nitrates.

Parsley: Contains a good amount of nitrates.

Cabbage: Both green and red cabbage contain nitrates.

Raspberries: Among the few fruits with high nitrate levels.

Strawberries: Among the few fruits with high nitrate levels.

FAT

Why We Need Fat

Warning! If you have specific dietary needs or conditions that affect your ability to eat particular types of food, consult a nutritionist before implementing my recommendations.

Fats are an essential part of a balanced diet. They provide your body with energy and support cell growth. They also help protect your organs and help keep your body warm. Fats also help your body absorb some nutrients and produce important hormones.

Steroid hormones are cholesterol-based molecules. Among these hormones are testosterone and estrogen. So, not eating enough healthy fat could reduce your testosterone levels.

However, not all fats are created equal. They are typically divided into four categories: saturated fats, trans fats, monounsaturated fats, and polyunsaturated fats.

Overview of Fats

Saturated Fats: These are usually solid at room temperature and come mainly from animal food sources, such as red meat, poultry, and full-fat dairy products. They raise total blood cholesterol levels and low-density lipoprotein (LDL) cholesterol levels, which can increase your risk of cardiovascular disease.

Trans Fats: These are created in an industrial process that adds hydrogen to liquid vegetable oils to make them more solid. They are often found in fried foods, bakery products, and margarine. Like saturated fats, trans fats can raise cholesterol levels in the blood, but they also lower 'good' high-density lipoprotein (HDL) cholesterol levels and increase the risk of heart disease.

Monounsaturated Fats: These are typically liquid at room temperature but start to solidify at cold temperatures. Monounsaturated fats can help reduce bad LDL cholesterol levels in your blood, lowering your risk of heart disease and stroke. They also provide nutrients to help develop and maintain your body's cells. Sources of monounsaturated fats include olive oil, canola oil, peanut oil, avocados, and most nuts.

Polyunsaturated Fats: These are also typically liquid at room temperature. They are found in plant-based foods and oils. Eating foods rich in polyunsaturated fats can help lower LDL cholesterol levels, reduce heart disease and stroke risk, and provide nutrients that help your cells function. They also provide essential fats that your body needs but can't produce independently. These essential fats must come from food. Foods rich in polyunsaturated fats include fatty fish like salmon, mackerel, and trout, and seeds like flaxseed and sunflower seeds, as well as walnuts and soybean oil.

In general, it's best to limit your intake of saturated fats and avoid trans fats as much as possible. A diet rich in monounsaturated and polyunsaturated fats can help promote better health. That being said, all fats are high in calories, so they should be consumed in moderation. Always strive for a balanced diet that includes a variety of foods from all food groups.

Here is a short list of sources of healthy fats

Avocado: Avocados are rich in monounsaturated fats, which can help lower bad cholesterol levels and reduce the risk of heart disease.

Olive Oil: Extra virgin olive oil is an excellent source of monounsaturated fats and is associated with numerous health benefits, including reducing inflammation and improving heart health.

Nuts and Seeds: Almonds, walnuts, flaxseeds, chia seeds, and hemp seeds are all packed with healthy fats, including omega-3 fatty acids. They are also a good source of fiber and other essential nutrients.

Fatty Fish: Salmon, mackerel, sardines, trout, and tuna are examples of fatty fish that contain omega-3 fatty acids, which are beneficial for heart health, brain function, and reducing inflammation.

Coconut Oil: While coconut oil is high in saturated fat, it consists mostly of medium-chain triglycerides (MCTs), which are metabolized differently by the body. MCTs are considered healthy fats and may benefit weight management and brain health.

Chia Seeds: Chia seeds are not only a great source of healthy fats but also rich in fiber, antioxidants, and other important nutrients. They can be added to smoothies or used as an egg substitute in baking.

Full-Fat Yogurt: Yogurt made from whole milk or full-fat dairy products contains healthy fats, protein, and probiotics that promote gut health.

Dark Chocolate: Dark chocolate with a high cocoa content (70% or more) contains healthy fats, fiber, and antioxidants. It should be consumed in moderation due to its calorie density.

Nut Butters: Natural nut butters, such as almond butter or peanut butter, provide healthy fats and can be spread on whole-grain toast or used as a dip for fruits and vegetables.

Seeds: Besides chia seeds, other seeds like sunflower seeds and pumpkin seeds are also good sources of healthy fats, fiber, and various vitamins and minerals.

PROTEIN

Why Protein is Important

Warning! If you have specific dietary needs or conditions that affect your ability to eat particular types of food, consult a nutritionist before implementing my recommendations.

Protein is one of the three major macronutrients found in food, the others being carbohydrates and fats. Proteins are complex molecules of amino acids linked together in long chains.

Proteins in food are used to replace and repair proteins in the body. When we eat proteins, our bodies break them down into amino acids, which are used to make new proteins.

Proteins play numerous critical roles in the body, including:

Growth and Maintenance: Protein is termed the body's building block. It is used to build and repair tissues, including muscle.

Enzymes: Many proteins act as enzymes, catalyzing biochemical reactions crucial in metabolism.

Hormones: Some proteins function as hormones, chemical messengers that help communicate information throughout the body. Insulin, for example, is a protein hormone.

Antibodies: Proteins also function as antibodies, which help the body defend against disease and illness.

Transport and Storage: Certain proteins help transport molecules throughout the body. Hemoglobin, for example, is a protein that carries oxygen from the lungs to the body's tissues.

Healthy Sources of Protein

Animal-Based Proteins:

- **Lean Meats:** These include chicken, turkey, and lean cuts of pork and beef. They're excellent protein sources, with the bonus of other nutrients like B vitamins and iron.

- **Fish:** Salmon, tuna, and mackerel are rich in protein and provide beneficial omega-3 fatty acids. Lighter fish like cod or haddock are also great sources of protein.

- **Eggs:** Eggs are one of the most complete protein sources available, containing all essential amino acids. They also provide a variety of vitamins and minerals.

- **Dairy:** Milk, cheese, and yogurt are good sources of protein. Choose low-fat or non-fat versions to limit your saturated fat intake.

Plant-Based Proteins:

- **Legumes:** Beans, peas, and lentils are protein-rich and provide dietary fiber.

- **Nuts and Seeds:** Almonds, peanuts, sunflower seeds, chia seeds, and flax seeds are high in protein and provide healthy fats and fiber.

- **Protein-Rich Vegetables:** Some vegetables, like spinach, broccoli, and peas, contain a good amount of protein relative to their calorie content.

Eat Organic

Unfortunately, eating quality food is relatively expensive. Just like with vegetables, eating organic meat is healthier. Also, like vegetables, it's not about the nutritional content. It's about avoiding chemicals that can harm your body.

What is Meant by Organic Meat?

The term commonly used for raising animals without antibiotics, hormones, or artificial additives and allowing them to engage in natural behaviors is "organic farming" or "organic production." When it comes to specific types of animals, the terms can vary slightly:

Cows: "Organic beef" refers to cattle raised on organic feed without the use of synthetic pesticides or fertilizers. They are also not treated with antibiotics or hormones.

Chickens: "Organic poultry" refers to chickens raised on organic feed without the use of synthetic pesticides or fertilizers. They are not treated with antibiotics or hormones and can access the outdoors.

Pigs: "Organic pork" refers to pigs raised on organic feed without the use of synthetic pesticides or fertilizers. They are not treated with antibiotics or hormones and can access the outdoors.

It's important to note that the specific regulations and standards for organic farming may vary between countries or regions. Certification bodies and governmental organizations often set guidelines for what can be labeled as organic in a particular jurisdiction.

Avoid Processed Meats

Even if you can afford organic meat, at least avoid processed meats. Processed meats are meat products that have undergone various processes to extend their shelf life, enhance flavor, or change their texture. These processes typically involve curing, smoking, salting, or adding preservatives.

Some common examples of processed meats:

- **Bacon:** Cured and smoked pork belly slices.

- **Sausages:** Ground meat mixed with spices, herbs, and other ingredients, typically encased in a casing.

- **Hot dogs:** A type of sausage made from a mixture of finely ground meat, often including pork, beef, or poultry, along with other additives and preservatives.

- **Deli meats or cold cuts:** Sliced meats, such as turkey, ham, roast beef, or salami, are often cured and processed for extended shelf life.

- **Pepperoni:** A type of cured and seasoned Italian sausage, usually made from pork or beef.

- **Ham:** Pork that has been cured, often by smoking or brining, and may be cooked or uncooked.

It's important to note that while processed meats can be

convenient and flavorful, they have been associated with certain health risks. Regularly consuming processed meats has been linked to an increased risk of chronic conditions like heart disease, certain cancers (particularly colorectal cancer), and other adverse health effects. It's generally recommended to consume processed meats in moderation and prioritize whole, unprocessed meats as part of a balanced diet.

JUNK FOOD

Why is Junk Food Addictive?

Warning! If you have specific dietary needs or conditions that affect your ability to eat particular types of food, consult a nutritionist before implementing my recommendations.

Getting people to give up food that they enjoy is very difficult. Food companies have engineered junk food to be addictive. Our hunter-gatherer ancestors lived in a world where available calories were limited. They developed cravings for fats and sweet items, driving them to pursue calorie-rich foods. We crave salt for a similar reason. Dietary salt was much more limited, and they needed adequate amounts in their diets.

Unfortunately, those cravings that served our ancestors well in a world of limited resources are being used by food companies to sell us food that tastes great but has no significant nutritional value.

What is Junk Food?

Junk food is often defined as food that is high in calories but low in nutritional value. There isn't a universally agreed upon, scientific definition of "junk food," but typically, the term is used to describe foods and beverages that are high in added sugars, saturated fat, and sodium and are often highly processed or ready-to-eat.

These might include items like:

- Fast food like hamburgers, hot dogs, and fried chicken.

- Sugary drinks like soda and energy drinks.

- High-sugar snacks like candies and cookies.

- High-fat snacks like potato chips and other fried snacks.

- Processed foods like ready-made meals and instant noodles.

These foods are low in fiber, protein, vitamins, and minerals, all important for maintaining a healthy body. Regularly consuming junk food can lead to health issues like obesity, heart disease, diabetes, and other serious conditions.

Cheat Days

Giving up these foods is an exercise in willpower for most people. Clearly, it would be best to give up junk food entirely. However, it may be more realistic to plan on allowing yourself to indulge occasionally.

One Day Per Week

Many diets incorporate "cheat days." The idea is to select times when you will allow yourself to eat and drink junk food. Usually, it's suggested that you select one day a week for indulging.

Indulging on Special Occasions

Here is my strategy:

- I go out to eat once or twice a month. I put my diet aside and order what I want on those occasions.

- When I'm traveling for any reason, I relax my diet. While I do my best, I don't worry about indulging a little.

- On special occasions, like family get-togethers, weddings, birthdays, etc. I forget my diet and eat what I want.

Whatever strategy you use, guard against too many cheat days. The important thing is that you cut back as much as possible on junk food.

WATER

You Need to Drink Water

Water is not complicated. You need to drink adequate amounts of water for your health, and most people don't drink enough. It is possible to drink too much water, but that's a very rare and unusual problem.

Fortunately, you can count most drinks like tea and coffee towards your water intake. Just avoid sugary drinks, and of course, alcohol does not count.

One of my favorite drinks:

16 ounces of water

Add 1 tablespoon of apple cider vinegar to the water

Squeeze 1/4 to 1/2 lemon into the water

Mix and drink!

Sources of Safe Water

Unfortunately, we can not count on tap water as a safe water supply. Of course, the water quality will vary greatly from community to community, but in general, it is a good idea to filter the water from your faucet.

Filters

There are many ways to filter your water. There are countertop systems you fill with water manually and water filter systems you can install into your plumbing. Of course, those are quite expensive and only practical if you own your property.

Bottled Water

Bottled water is another alternative. Unfortunately, most bottled water comes in plastic bottles. Plastic is filled with estrogenic chemicals that can, among other things, lower testosterone levels in men and cause infertility in men and women. If you drink bottled water, drink water that comes in glass or metal containers.

Resources:

How to calculate the amount of water you need -

https://www.umsystem.edu/totalrewards/wellness/how-to-calculate-how-much-water-you-should-drink

Countertop water filters -

https://www.drinking-water.org/filter/best/countertop/

CHAPTER SIX

Mental Toughness

MENTAL TOUGHNESS

"I don't stop when I'm tired. I stop when I'm done." –
David Goggins.

"Nothing can stop the man with the right mental
attitude from achieving his goal; nothing on earth
can help the man with the wrong mental attitude." –
Thomas Jefferson.

"In terms of instilling the values of mental
toughness and work ethic, discipline is the gift that
keeps on giving." – **William Baldwin.**

What is Mental Toughness?

Metal toughness can be hard to define, but generally, it describes
the ability and willingness to persevere and keep on task despite any
discomfort, pain, fatigue, or frustration.

Mental Toughness and Endurance Exercise

Endurance exercises like rucking can help build mental toughness

Until someone becomes properly conditioned, endurance exercise
is uncomfortable. Getting in shape requires setting a goal and
incrementally pushing oneself past one's comfort zone. The more one
pushes themselves outside of their comfort zone, the more comfortable
they will become with discomfort.

The act of pushing oneself to reach goals that are uncomfortable and difficult is an act of discipline necessary for building mental toughness. Of course, there is much more to building mental toughness than pushing oneself physically. However, it is an important part of a much bigger picture.

CHAPTER SEVEN

Communication Skills

COMMUNICATION SKILLS

If you are out rucking alone or with a group, it's essential to have the ability to get help if you are injured or lost. In a group, it is necessary to communicate with each other about the route, safety procedures, and preventing people from getting lost.

Whether alone or in a group, it's always a good idea to let someone know and trust where you are going and when you expect to return or check in with them. This is especially true if you are rucking on your own.

When rucking in a group, everyone should have a cell phone, and everyone in the group should have each other's numbers in their contacts. It's also an excellent idea to turn on tracking functions, at least while you are out rucking.

Using a cell phone will simplify group and emergency communications. **Unfortunately, relying on cell phones or walkie-talkies is a terrible idea. Electronics are fragile and unreliable. Always have a backup plan.**

The Downside of Cell Phones:

- They need to be kept charged, and if you don't have a way to recharge your phone, it's useless for communication.

- They break easily. Most cell phones are not designed for ruggedness. They are vulnerable to breaking if dropped or exposed to water.

- They can overheat if it's too hot.

- They need a signal. This will probably not be an issue in urban or suburban areas, but cell phone reception can be spotty or nonexistent in the wilderness or the countryside.

The bottom line is to use your cell phone if you can, but don't depend on it in an emergency.

Learn Emergency Signals:

Knowledge of using visual and auditory signals to communicate distress or call for help in an emergency. This includes using whistles, mirrors, flashlights, reflective devices, or natural materials to create visible signals.

Everyone should have the following with them for emergency signaling.

- A loud whistle

- A small mirror or reflective device

- A brightly colored cloth or t-shirt that is easily visible

- A flashlight

- Something reflective that can be seen when a light shines on it in the dark.

- Glow sticks

Briefing and Debriefing:

Conduct thorough briefings before setting out on a day's trek and debriefings at the end. This involves discussing the route, potential hazards, the weather forecast, and emergency plans.

Establish a Route and Rally Points:

- Before heading out, everyone should discuss the route and rally points.
- Each person should have a paper map with the route marked on it.
- Make sure everyone understands the root and how to read the map.

Rally points are locations along the route to head to if the group is separated. If separated from your group, you can backtrack to the nearest rally point and wait. Once the other group members realize you are missing, they can return to previous rally points to find you.

Check-ins:

Establish check-in routines with your group to ensure everyone is accounted for and to assess everyone's condition, energy levels, and hydration status. This can help make informed decisions about pace, breaks, and whether to continue or turn back.

Do regular check-ins with everyone at each rally point. Check-ins can be done more regularly as needed. It is vitally essential everyone is accounted for at each rally point. So once someone is missing, it is noticed quickly, and the group can backtrack to the previous rally point to find them.

You can call someone you trust and check in with them if you are alone. If something should happen to you, the more information they have the easier it will be to find you.

If You Are Lost:

If you are completely lost and do not know how to find the rally points. Stop where you are. The more you walk at this point, the more lost you are likely to get. Attempt to make yourself easier to find by waiting in a relatively clear area and using emergency signals.

If You Are Injured:

If you are injured and cannot make it to a rallying point. Wait where you are, attempt to make yourself as visible as possible, and start emergency signaling methods if possible.

CHAPTER EIGHT

Terrain Navigation and Route Planning

NAVIGATION AND ROUTE PLANNING

Land navigation is a big subject. It's much too big to cover thoroughly in this book. So, this chapter aims to introduce you to the skills needed for map reading and land navigation. I recommend getting the Army manual **Map Reading And Land Navigation - FM 3-25.26 US Army Field Manual** or a comparable land navigation book. I also recommend looking for someone who can teach you the fundamentals.

Generally, if you are rucking in urban or suburban areas or sticking to trails, you will need a map with the roads and trails, a way to orient the map, and probably not much more. Map reading is an essential but often overlooked skill if you are going off-trail. It is also necessary to practice these skills in a controlled environment before trying them out in the field. **Getting lost in the wilderness can quickly become a life-and-death situation.**

Map Reading and Land Navigation Skills

Understanding Map Symbols and Scales: Familiarize yourself with your map's symbols, terrain features, and scale. This will help you interpret the map correctly. Maps used for land navigation have a standard way of representing things on a map.

Orienting the Map: Use your compass to align the map with magnetic north, and then learn how to make the proper adjustments to align the map to true north and grid north. This ensures the map's orientation matches the actual landscape.

Identifying Landmarks: To help determine your current location, look for prominent features in the environment that are also visible on the map, such as hills, rivers, and buildings.

Taking a Bearing: Use your compass to determine the direction from your current position to your destination. This is called taking a bearing.

Transferring Bearings to the Map: Place the edge of the compass on the map, aligning one end with your current location and the other with your destination. Rotate the compass housing until the north lines on the compass align with the map's north. This gives you the map bearing.

Following a Bearing in the Field: Align the compass so the needle matches the bearing you've set. Then, look ahead to identify a feature in the distance that aligns with your bearing and walk towards it. Repeat this process to stay on course.

Pacing and Timing: Estimate distances by counting steps or using time. Knowing your pace count for a specific distance helps track how far you've traveled. To determine your pace count, you must count your paces over a known distance, like 100 meters of similar terrain. You can then determine the approximate distance you have traveled according to your pace count.

Using Handrails and Catching Features: A handrail is a feature that leads in the direction you're traveling, like a river or trail. A catching feature is something that, if you see it, you have gone too far. It can be any feature, such as a road or coastline but reasonably close to your target. By identifying catch features, you can prevent yourself from overshooting your target too far. If you hit a catch feature, you know that you have to backtrack.

Re-Section and Triangulation: If you're unsure of your location, you can use these methods to find it. Re-section involves taking bearings from your location to two or three known points on the map. Triangulation is similar but involves taking bearings from known points to your location.

Contour Lines: Learn how to read contour lines on the map to understand the terrain, including identifying hills, valleys, ridges, and depressions. Contour lines on a map represent lines of equal elevation, indicating the terrain's height and shape. The spacing and pattern of these lines reveal features such as hills, valleys, and slopes.

CHAPTER NINE

Emergency Procedures and Safety

EMERGENCY PROCEDURES AND SAFETY

Planning

Always plan as if something will go wrong. It's better to be prepared for something that never happens than to be unprepared when something does happen. Of course, you can't be prepared for every possible contingency, but you can be prepared for most of the problems you will likely encounter. Fortunately, it's not very difficult to plan ahead. So, let's go over the basics.

Communication

This is the single most important part of planning. It is so important that I devoted a whole chapter to it. Please review the Chapter Seven chapter. **Remember, do not depend on your cell phone!**

First Aid

Have a first aid kit. Your kit should have what you need to treat the most likely issues you will encounter. Remember that every environment poses different threats. For example, where I live in New England, dealing with a snake bite is unlikely. However, if you are rucking in the desert, the chances of a snake bite increase dramatically.

Consider the types of threats your environment poses and stock your kit accordingly. For instance, I wouldn't pack a snake-bite kit if I were rucking close to my home, but I would if I were rucking in an area with poisonous snakes.

If you or someone in your group has ailments or conditions that may require immediate intervention, you should definitely have everything on hand to deal with them. Examples might be Asma, allergies, or diabetes. Of course, there are many other possibilities; the point is to know what they are before going out and being properly prepared.

Regardless of the environment, there are common injuries for which you should be prepared.

- **Blisters:** Caused by friction, leading to painful, fluid-filled sacs on the skin.

- **Cuts and Scrapes:** From falls or brushing against rough vegetation.

- **Sprains and Strains:** Twisting or pulling muscles and ligaments, especially in ankles and knees.

- **Tick Bites:** Ticks can attach to any part of the human body and are often found in warm, moist areas.

- **Insect Stings:** Bees, wasps, and other insects can sting, causing pain, swelling, and allergic reactions.

- **Sunburn:** Extended exposure to the sun without adequate protection can lead to sunburn.

You can have the best first aid kit in the world, but it's not very useful if you don't know what to do with it. **If you are not well versed in first aid, take some first aid courses.** Even if you never go rucking, it's always a good idea to be trained in first aid. I consider it a basic life skill that most people ignore.

Environmental Emergencies

Each environment can pose unique safety issues. Below are some common environmental hazards.

Heat Exhaustion: Caused by dehydration and excessive sweating without enough fluid intake.

Dehydration: Insufficient water intake, especially in hot weather or during strenuous activity.

Hypothermia: Occurs in cold conditions when the body loses heat faster than it can produce it.

Equipment for Environmental Hazards

Water: Always have enough water on you, especially when it's hot. The problem with water is that it is quite heavy. If it is impractical to carry enough water, I recommend carrying personal water filters with you and planning your route to stop at safe water sources for resupply. Obviously, use and test the water filters before you need to use them.

Extra Clothing: When you go out, you should assume something will go wrong, forcing you to stop and stay put. Depending on the range of temperatures you can encounter in your environment, you should have extra layers to stay warm. Take extra underwear and socks. If your underwear and socks are wet from perspiration and sweating in a cold environment, that could lead to hypothermia.

Emergency Poncho: A mylar emergency poncho is light, cheap, and easy to carry. If you are in an area where rain is possible, this item can keep you and your equipment dry and prevent hypothermia.

Emergency Bivy Sack: A Bivy sack is a lightweight, waterproof shelter that protects users from the elements. If you will be stuck where you are for a while, a Mylar Bivy sack could be a lifesaver. Mylar bivy sacks are cheap and lightweight, and they can dramatically increase your chances of survival in cold and/or wet weather. **Putting one in your pack should be a no-brainer.**

General Purpose Emergency Items

Some general-purpose items will come in handy in emergencies. If you are into bushcraft or survival, you will likely know where I'm going with this list. This is a minimalist list of items that could greatly increase your chances of survival.

Multitools: A good multitool has a million uses. Be sure to choose a multitool based on what you will likely need it for. If you are going out into the wilderness, a multitool with screwdrivers may not be as useful as a multi-tool with scissors and a saw. My point is not to pick just any multitool; pick one that will serve you best in the environment you are rucking in.

Cordage: Cordage is just one of those things you take for granted until you need it. I recommend Paracord or bank line cordage.

Gorilla Tape: Like cordage, people don't think about this until they need it. Gorilla tape has many uses. Among those uses, it can be used as an emergency bandage and as a tinder for starting a fire.

Metal containers: At least one of your canteens should be a single wall metal container. If you have to, you can use it to boil water to make it safe to drink. Of course, this would require a fire, so if you don't know how to start a fire safely (most people don't), opt for high-quality water filters.

Bic Lighter: Most people lack the skills to start a fire without matches or a lighter. Those skills can take time to learn and master. So, I recommend having a Bic Lighter on you at all times, along with something that can be used for tinder, like Gorilla Tape.

Large Bandanna: A piece of cotton cloth has many uses, from a makeshift hat to a bandage or a water strainer before boiling it.

CHAPTER TEN

Environmental Stewardship

ENVIRONMENTAL STEWARDSHIP

Whenever I go rucking or spend time in the wilderness, I always see the tell-tale signs of selfish people who don't respect nature. Their trash is everywhere. Typically I find cans, paper trash, and bags of dog poop. Sometimes, I find discarded clothing. I've even found insulators for high-voltage electrical wires. These insulators are big, heavy ceramic components. Someone lugged these things out into the forest a left them there. Why anyone would do that is beyond me.

I always try to take a trash bag with me when I go out into nature. When I can, I pick up the trash, I find. All too often, I leave with a full bag. Please don't be that guy (or girl). To the best of your ability, clean up after yourself and follow the guidelines below. These principles aim to ensure that natural places are pristine and enjoyable for future generations.

Leave No Trace Guidelines

Leave No Trace is a set of outdoor ethics promoting conservation. It consists of principles designed to guide behavior for the responsible use of natural areas to minimize human impact. The seven principles are:

Plan Ahead and Prepare: Proper planning can help minimize the impact on natural resources by considering travel time, regulations, safety precautions, and goals.

Travel and Camp on Durable Surfaces: Avoid damaging vegetation and soil by sticking to established trails and camping sites.

Dispose of Waste Properly: Pack out all trash, leftover food, and litter. Use toilet facilities or, if unavailable, bury human waste properly.

Leave What You Find: Preserve the past and natural conditions by not taking cultural or natural objects, and avoid altering sites.

Minimize Campfire Impacts: Use a lightweight stove for cooking and enjoy campfires in established fire rings, if at all, to minimize damage.

Respect Wildlife: Observe wildlife from a distance without feeding them or affecting their behavior.

Be Considerate of Other Visitors: Ensure the outdoors remains a quiet, enjoyable space for all visitors by being respectful and courteous.

CHAPTER ELEVEN

Final Thoughts

FINAL THOUGHTS

This book contains a lot of information about rucking, but don't overcomplicate things. Get a backpack, put a few pounds in it, and start walking. Like any other type of exercise, start out easy and build up gradually.

Rucking can be a great way to improve your fitness. You can do it as your sole form of exercise or as part of a broader fitness program. The important thing is that you get out and move.

Once you start rucking, refine your technique and adjust your equipment over time. You don't need a special pack to start. However, you will probably want to invest in a well-designed pack as you start going further, faster, and with more weight.

Keep safety in mind at all times, especially if you are going to be rucking in isolated areas. Even if you are a few yards from the nearest road or building, if you are injured, your cell phone isn't working, no one can see you, and no one knows where you are, then you could be in serious trouble. It's not uncommon for people to go out on a hike, get hurt or lost, and die from exposure because they were unprepared for the temperature drop once the sun went down. Don't be that person. Planning ahead can prevent this from happening.

If you want to explore rucking in more depth or feel you need some coaching, please contact **Michael Glover** or **Ken Schafer**. Our contact information is below.

Michael Glover - theartofrucking@gmail.com

Website: www.theartofrucking.com

Ken Schafer - contact@healthysexualitywithken.com

Website: www.healthysexualitywithken.com

Now, go hit some trails!

Made in the USA
Coppell, TX
06 June 2024

33215034R00079